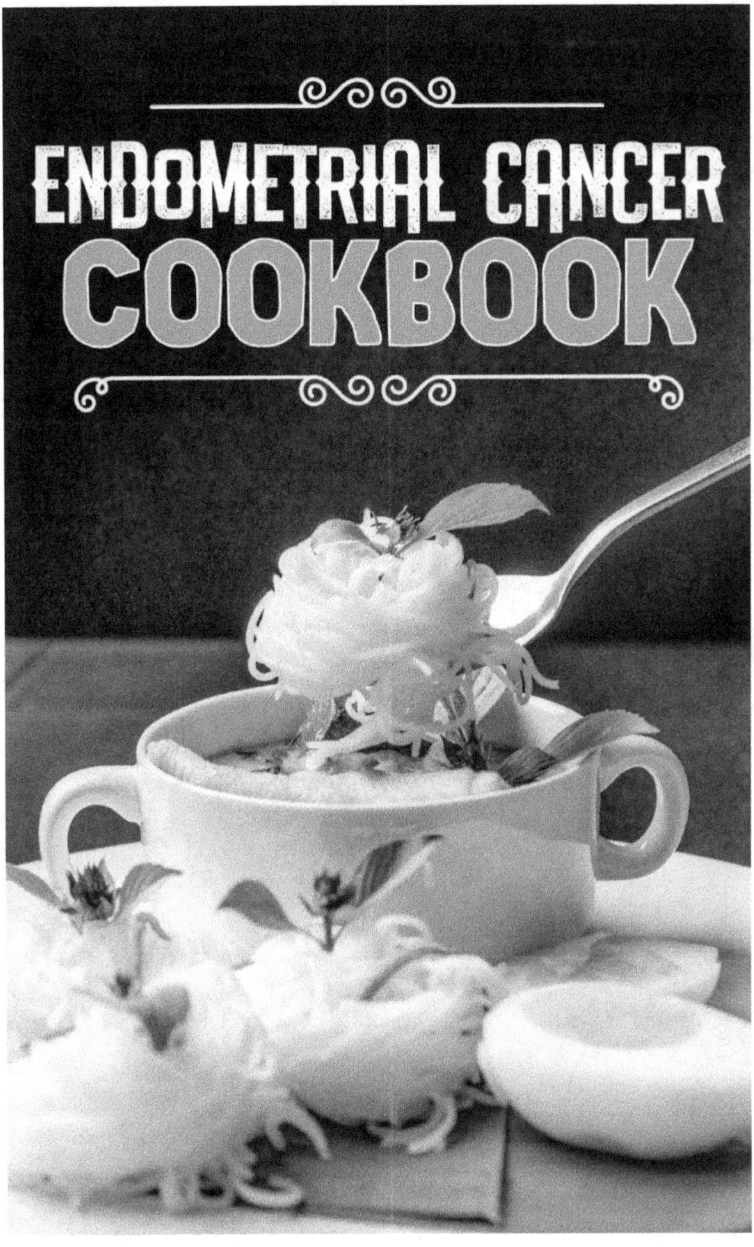

ENDOMETRIAL CANCER COOKBOOK

This book belongs to...

Endometrial Cancer Cookbook

Recipes to Nourish and Boost Health

-- Drusilla Ronnell Allison --

Attribution

This cover was designed with help from pexels.com

ISBN

9798323629718

Imprint

Independently Published

== Disclaimer ==

The information contained in this book is for general informational purposes only. The author and publisher have made every effort to ensure that the content provided is accurate and up-to-date at the time of publication. However, medical knowledge is constantly evolving, and individual circumstances vary. Therefore, the author and publisher do not make any representations or warranties of any kind, express or implied, about the completeness, accuracy, reliability, suitability, or availability of the information contained in this book.

The information provided is not a substitute for professional medical advice, diagnosis, or treatment. Always seek the advice of your physician or another qualified healthcare provider with any questions you may have regarding a medical condition. Never disregard professional medical advice or delay seeking it because of something you have read in this book.

The author and publisher disclaim any responsibility for any adverse effects resulting directly or indirectly from the use of the information provided in this book. The reader assumes full responsibility for consulting a qualified healthcare professional regarding health conditions and before starting any new treatment or making changes to existing treatment.

The inclusion of specific products, services, or medical procedures in this book does not imply endorsement. The author and publisher shall have no liability for any damages or loss arising out of, or in connection with, the use of this book.

It is recommended to independently verify any information provided in this book and consult with a qualified healthcare professional for advice tailored to your individual circumstances.

List of Contents

Personal Note for This Cookbook

As you embark on your journey to nourish and boost your health during and after cancer treatment, remember that each recipe in this cookbook is crafted with care and intention. Whether you're seeking comfort, nourishment, or a burst of flavor, I hope these dishes provide you with the sustenance and joy you deserve.

Throughout the ups and downs of your journey, may you find solace in the kitchen, creating meals that not only fuel your body but also nurture your spirit. Remember to listen to your body, honor your cravings, and savor each bite with gratitude.

Important note about this book: Please note that the information provided here is for general knowledge and should not replace professional medical advice. If you have specific concerns or questions about **Endometrial Cancer**, it's best to consult with a healthcare professional familiar with your medical history.

1. Introduction

Welcome to the Endometrial Cancer Cookbook, a collection of nourishing and comforting recipes designed to support your health during and after treatment. Endometrial cancer can present unique challenges, but through mindful eating and nourishing ingredients, we can cultivate strength, resilience, and well-being.

This cookbook is more than just a collection of recipes; it's a journey toward healing and empowerment. Each dish has been thoughtfully crafted to provide essential nutrients, promote healing, and bring joy to your table. From comforting soups to vibrant salads, hearty mains to wholesome snacks, these recipes offer a variety of flavors and textures to suit your palate and nutritional needs.

Navigating a cancer diagnosis can be overwhelming, but finding solace in the kitchen can be a source of comfort and empowerment. As you explore these recipes, I encourage you to embrace the therapeutic power of cooking and nourish both your body and spirit.

Whether you're seeking recipes to soothe side effects, boost energy levels, or simply enjoy a delicious meal with loved ones, this cookbook is here to support you every step of the way. Let the aroma of simmering soups, the sizzle of grilled vegetables, and the sweetness of baked treats fill your kitchen with warmth and healing.

Remember, food is not only fuel for the body but also nourishment for the soul. May these recipes bring you comfort, nourishment, and moments of culinary joy as you journey toward wellness.

2. Immune-Boosting Vegetable Soup

Ingredients:

- 1 tablespoon olive oil
- 1 onion, diced
- 2 cloves garlic, minced
- 4 carrots, sliced
- 2 stalks celery, chopped
- 1 sweet potato, diced
- 1 zucchini, sliced
- 6 cups vegetable broth
- 1 teaspoon turmeric
- 1 teaspoon ginger, grated
- Salt and pepper to taste
- Fresh parsley for garnish

Instructions:

1. Heat olive oil in a large pot over medium heat. Add diced onion and minced garlic, sauté until fragrant.

2. Add sliced carrots, chopped celery, diced sweet potato, and sliced zucchini to the pot. Cook for 5 minutes, stirring occasionally.

3. Pour in vegetable broth and bring to a boil. Reduce heat and simmer for 15-20 minutes or until vegetables are tender.

4. Stir in turmeric, grated ginger, salt, and pepper. Adjust seasoning according to taste.

5. Serve hot, garnished with fresh parsley.

3. Protein-Packed Quinoa Salad

Ingredients:

- 1 cup quinoa, rinsed

- 2 cups water

- 1 can chickpeas, drained and rinsed

- 1 cucumber, diced

- 1 bell pepper, diced

- 1/4 cup red onion, finely chopped

- 1/4 cup fresh parsley, chopped

- 1/4 cup olive oil

- 2 tablespoons lemon juice

- 1 teaspoon honey

- Salt and pepper to taste

Instructions:

1. In a medium saucepan, bring water to a boil. Add quinoa, reduce heat, cover, and simmer for 15 minutes or until water is absorbed and quinoa is cooked. Remove from heat and let it cool.

2. In a large bowl, combine cooked quinoa, chickpeas, diced cucumber, diced bell pepper, chopped red onion, and chopped parsley.

3. In a small bowl, whisk together olive oil, lemon juice, honey, salt, and pepper to make the dressing.

4. Pour the dressing over the quinoa salad and toss until well combined.

5. Chill in the refrigerator for at least 30 minutes before serving.

4. Berry Blast Smoothie

Ingredients:

- 1 cup mixed berries (strawberries, blueberries, raspberries)
- 1 banana
- 1 cup spinach leaves
- 1/2 cup Greek yogurt
- 1/2 cup almond milk
- 1 tablespoon honey (optional)
- Ice cubes

Instructions:

1. Place mixed berries, banana, spinach leaves, Greek yogurt, almond milk, and honey (if using) in a blender.
2. Blend until smooth and creamy.
3. Add ice cubes and blend again until desired consistency is reached.
4. Pour into glasses and serve immediately.

5. Nutrient-Rich Avocado Toast

Ingredients:

- 2 slices whole grain bread

- 1 ripe avocado

- 1 tablespoon lemon juice

- Salt and pepper to taste

- Optional toppings: sliced tomato, sprouts, poached egg, smoked salmon

Instructions:

1. Toast the slices of whole grain bread until golden brown.

2. In a small bowl, mash the ripe avocado with lemon juice, salt, and pepper until smooth.

3. Spread the mashed avocado evenly onto the toasted bread slices.

4. Add optional toppings such as sliced tomato, sprouts, poached egg, or smoked salmon as desired.

5. Serve immediately for a delicious and nutrient-packed meal.

6. Healing Turmeric Golden Milk

Ingredients:

- 2 cups unsweetened almond milk
- 1 teaspoon ground turmeric
- 1/2 teaspoon ground cinnamon
- 1/4 teaspoon ground ginger
- Pinch of black pepper
- 1 tablespoon honey or maple syrup (optional)
- 1 teaspoon coconut oil (optional)

Instructions:

1. In a small saucepan, heat almond milk over medium heat until warmed but not boiling.

2. Whisk in ground turmeric, ground cinnamon, ground ginger, black pepper, and honey or maple syrup if using.

3. Continue to whisk until all ingredients are well combined and the milk is heated through.

4. Remove from heat and stir in coconut oil if desired for added creaminess.

5. Pour into mugs and enjoy this comforting and healing beverage.

7. Energizing Green Smoothie Bowl

Ingredients:

- 2 cups spinach leaves

- 1 ripe banana, frozen

- 1/2 avocado

- 1/2 cup pineapple chunks, frozen

- 1/2 cup almond milk

- Toppings: sliced banana, fresh berries, granola, chia seeds, coconut flakes

Instructions:

1. In a blender, combine spinach leaves, frozen banana, avocado, frozen pineapple chunks, and almond milk.

2. Blend until smooth and creamy, adding more almond milk if needed to reach desired consistency.

3. Pour the green smoothie into a bowl.

4. Top with sliced banana, fresh berries, granola, chia seeds, and coconut flakes for added texture and flavor.

5. Enjoy this refreshing and nutrient-packed smoothie bowl for a satisfying meal or snack.

8. Roasted Vegetable Quinoa Bowl

Ingredients:

- 1 cup quinoa, rinsed

- 2 cups water or vegetable broth

- 2 cups mixed vegetables (such as broccoli, cauliflower, bell peppers, and cherry tomatoes), chopped

- 2 tablespoons olive oil

- 2 cloves garlic, minced

- 1 teaspoon dried herbs (such as thyme, rosemary, or oregano)

- Salt and pepper to taste

- Optional toppings: crumbled feta cheese, toasted nuts or seeds, avocado slices

Instructions:

1. Preheat the oven to 400°F (200°C). Line a baking sheet with parchment paper.

2. In a saucepan, bring water or vegetable broth to a boil. Add quinoa, reduce heat, cover, and simmer for 15 minutes or until quinoa is cooked and liquid is absorbed. Remove from heat and fluff with a fork.

3. In a large bowl, toss chopped mixed vegetables with olive oil, minced garlic, dried herbs, salt, and pepper until evenly coated.

4. Spread the seasoned vegetables in a single layer on the prepared baking sheet. Roast in the preheated oven for 20-25 minutes or until vegetables are tender and lightly browned, stirring halfway through.

5. Divide cooked quinoa among serving bowls and top with roasted vegetables.

6. Garnish with optional toppings such as crumbled feta cheese, toasted nuts or seeds, and avocado slices if desired.

7. Serve warm and enjoy this flavorful and nourishing quinoa bowl.

9. Creamy Butternut Squash Soup

Ingredients:

- 1 medium butternut squash, peeled, seeded, and diced
- 1 onion, diced
- 2 cloves garlic, minced
- 2 carrots, chopped
- 4 cups vegetable broth
- 1 teaspoon ground cumin
- 1/2 teaspoon ground nutmeg
- Salt and pepper to taste
- 1/2 cup coconut milk
- Fresh cilantro for garnish (optional)

Instructions:

1. In a large pot, combine diced butternut squash, diced onion, minced garlic, chopped carrots, and vegetable broth.

2. Bring the mixture to a boil, then reduce heat and simmer for 20-25 minutes or until vegetables are tender.

3. Using an immersion blender or transferring the mixture to a blender, puree until smooth.

4. Stir in ground cumin, ground nutmeg, salt, and pepper.

5. Add coconut milk and stir until well combined and heated through.

6. Taste and adjust seasoning if necessary.

7. Serve hot, garnished with fresh cilantro if desired.

10.Protein-Packed Lentil Salad

Ingredients:

- 1 cup dried green lentils

- 3 cups water or vegetable broth

- 1 cucumber, diced

- 1 bell pepper, diced

- 1/4 cup red onion, finely chopped

- 1/4 cup fresh parsley, chopped

- 2 tablespoons olive oil

- 2 tablespoons lemon juice

- 1 teaspoon Dijon mustard

- Salt and pepper to taste

Instructions:

1. Rinse the dried green lentils under cold water.

2. In a saucepan, combine rinsed lentils and water or vegetable broth. Bring to a boil, then reduce heat and simmer for 20-25 minutes or until lentils are tender.

3. Drain any excess liquid from the cooked lentils and let them cool slightly.

4. In a large bowl, combine cooked lentils, diced cucumber, diced bell pepper, chopped red onion, and chopped parsley.

5. In a small bowl, whisk together olive oil, lemon juice, Dijon mustard, salt, and pepper to make the dressing.

6. Pour the dressing over the lentil salad and toss until well combined.

7. Chill in the refrigerator for at least 30 minutes before serving.

11.Baked Salmon with Herb Crust

Ingredients:

- 4 salmon fillets

- 2 tablespoons olive oil

- 1 tablespoon Dijon mustard

- 1/4 cup breadcrumbs (use whole grain for added fiber)

- 2 tablespoons fresh parsley, chopped

- 1 tablespoon fresh dill, chopped

- 1 tablespoon fresh chives, chopped

- Salt and pepper to taste

- Lemon wedges for serving

Instructions:

1. Preheat the oven to 400°F (200°C). Line a baking sheet with parchment paper.

2. In a small bowl, mix together olive oil and Dijon mustard.

3. Place salmon fillets on the prepared baking sheet. Brush the tops of the fillets with the olive oil and mustard mixture.

4. In another bowl, combine breadcrumbs, chopped parsley, chopped dill, chopped chives, salt, and pepper.

5. Press the breadcrumb mixture onto the top of each salmon fillet, coating evenly.

6. Bake in the preheated oven for 12-15 minutes or until salmon is cooked through and the crust is golden brown.

7. Serve hot with lemon wedges on the side.

12. Turmeric-Ginger Tea

Ingredients:

- 2 cups water

- 1-inch piece of fresh ginger, thinly sliced

- 1 teaspoon ground turmeric

- 1 tablespoon honey

- Juice of half a lemon

Instructions:

1. In a small saucepan, bring water to a boil.

2. Add thinly sliced ginger and ground turmeric to the boiling water.

3. Reduce heat and simmer for 5 minutes.

4. Remove from heat and strain the tea into cups.

5. Stir in honey and lemon juice.

6. Serve hot and enjoy the soothing and immune-boosting benefits of this turmeric-ginger tea.

13.Quinoa Stuffed Bell Peppers

Ingredients:

- 4 large bell peppers, any color

- 1 cup quinoa, rinsed

- 2 cups vegetable broth

- 1 tablespoon olive oil

- 1 onion, diced

- 2 cloves garlic, minced

- 1 zucchini, diced

- 1 cup cherry tomatoes, halved

- 1 cup cooked black beans

- 1 teaspoon ground cumin

- 1 teaspoon paprika

- Salt and pepper to taste

- 1/4 cup chopped fresh cilantro

- Optional: shredded cheese for topping

Instructions:

1. Preheat the oven to 375°F (190°C). Grease a baking dish.

2. Cut the tops off the bell peppers and remove the seeds and membranes. Place the peppers in the prepared baking dish, cut side up.

3. In a saucepan, combine quinoa and vegetable broth. Bring to a boil, then reduce heat, cover, and simmer for 15-20 minutes or until quinoa is cooked and liquid is absorbed.

4. In a large skillet, heat olive oil over medium heat. Add diced onion and minced garlic, sauté until softened.

5. Add diced zucchini, halved cherry tomatoes, cooked black beans, ground cumin, paprika, salt, and pepper to the skillet. Cook for 5-7 minutes or until vegetables are tender.

6. Stir in cooked quinoa and chopped fresh cilantro until well combined.

7. Spoon the quinoa mixture into the prepared bell peppers, filling them evenly.

8. Optional: Sprinkle shredded cheese on top of each stuffed pepper.

9. Cover the baking dish with foil and bake in the preheated oven for 25-30 minutes or until the peppers are tender.

10. Serve hot and enjoy these flavorful and nutritious quinoa stuffed bell peppers.

14.Immune-Boosting Citrus Salad

Ingredients:

- 4 cups mixed salad greens (such as spinach, arugula, and kale)

- 2 oranges, peeled and sliced

- 1 grapefruit, peeled and segmented

- 1 avocado, sliced

- 1/4 cup sliced red onion

- 1/4 cup toasted walnuts or almonds

- 2 tablespoons extra virgin olive oil

- 1 tablespoon balsamic vinegar

- Salt and pepper to taste

Instructions:

1. In a large bowl, combine mixed salad greens, sliced oranges, segmented grapefruit, sliced avocado, sliced red onion, and toasted walnuts or almonds.

2. In a small bowl, whisk together extra virgin olive oil, balsamic vinegar, salt, and pepper to make the dressing.

3. Drizzle the dressing over the salad and toss gently to coat.

4. Serve immediately as a refreshing and immune-boosting salad option.

15. Mediterranean Chickpea Salad

Ingredients:

- 2 cans (15 ounces each) chickpeas, drained and rinsed
- 1 cucumber, diced
- 1 bell pepper, diced
- 1 cup cherry tomatoes, halved
- 1/4 cup red onion, finely chopped
- 1/4 cup Kalamata olives, sliced
- 1/4 cup crumbled feta cheese
- 2 tablespoons chopped fresh parsley
- 2 tablespoons extra virgin olive oil
- 1 tablespoon red wine vinegar
- 1 teaspoon dried oregano
- Salt and pepper to taste

Instructions:

1. In a large bowl, combine chickpeas, diced cucumber, diced bell pepper, halved cherry tomatoes, chopped red onion, sliced Kalamata olives, crumbled feta cheese, and chopped fresh parsley.

2. In a small bowl, whisk together extra virgin olive oil, red wine vinegar, dried oregano, salt, and pepper to make the dressing.

3. Pour the dressing over the chickpea salad and toss gently to coat.

4. Serve chilled or at room temperature as a satisfying and flavorful salad option.

16. Coconut Chia Pudding

Ingredients:

- 1/4 cup chia seeds

- 1 cup coconut milk

- 1 tablespoon honey or maple syrup

- 1/2 teaspoon vanilla extract

- Optional toppings: sliced bananas, berries, shredded coconut, chopped nuts

Instructions:

1. In a bowl, combine chia seeds, coconut milk, honey or maple syrup, and vanilla extract.

2. Stir well to combine and make sure chia seeds are evenly distributed.

3. Cover the bowl and refrigerate for at least 4 hours or overnight, stirring occasionally to prevent clumping.

4. Once the mixture has thickened to a pudding-like consistency, divide it into serving cups or jars.

5. Top with sliced bananas, berries, shredded coconut, chopped nuts, or your favorite toppings.

6. Serve chilled and enjoy this creamy and nutritious coconut chia pudding as a healthy dessert or snack option.

17.Berry and Spinach Salad with Balsamic Vinaigrette

Ingredients:

- 4 cups baby spinach leaves

- 1 cup mixed berries (such as strawberries, blueberries, raspberries)

- 1/4 cup crumbled goat cheese

- 1/4 cup toasted pecans or walnuts

- 2 tablespoons balsamic vinegar

- 1 tablespoon extra virgin olive oil

- 1 teaspoon honey

- Salt and pepper to taste

Instructions:

1. In a large bowl, combine baby spinach leaves, mixed berries, crumbled goat cheese, and toasted pecans or walnuts.

2. In a small bowl, whisk together balsamic vinegar, extra virgin olive oil, honey, salt, and pepper to make the dressing.

3. Drizzle the dressing over the salad and toss gently to coat.

4. Serve immediately as a refreshing and nutritious salad option.

18.Oven-Roasted Brussels Sprouts

Ingredients:

- 1 pound Brussels sprouts, trimmed and halved
- 2 tablespoons olive oil
- 2 cloves garlic, minced
- 1 teaspoon dried thyme
- Salt and pepper to taste
- Optional: grated Parmesan cheese

Instructions:

1. Preheat the oven to 400°F (200°C). Line a baking sheet with parchment paper.
2. In a large bowl, toss halved Brussels sprouts with olive oil, minced garlic, dried thyme, salt, and pepper until evenly coated.
3. Spread the Brussels sprouts in a single layer on the prepared baking sheet.
4. Roast in the preheated oven for 20-25 minutes or until Brussels sprouts are tender and caramelized, stirring halfway through.
5. Optional: Sprinkle grated Parmesan cheese over the roasted Brussels sprouts before serving.
6. Serve hot as a flavorful and nutritious side dish.

19.Ginger-Turmeric Carrot Soup

Ingredients:

- 1 tablespoon olive oil

- 1 onion, diced

- 2 cloves garlic, minced

- 1 tablespoon fresh ginger, grated

- 1 tablespoon fresh turmeric, grated (or 1 teaspoon ground turmeric)

- 4 cups carrots, chopped

- 4 cups vegetable broth

- Salt and pepper to taste

- Optional toppings: plain yogurt, fresh cilantro, toasted pumpkin seeds

Instructions:

1. In a large pot, heat olive oil over medium heat. Add diced onion and minced garlic, sauté until softened.

2. Add grated ginger and grated turmeric to the pot, stir for 1-2 minutes until fragrant.

3. Add chopped carrots and vegetable broth to the pot. Bring to a boil, then reduce heat and simmer for 20-25 minutes or until carrots are tender.

4. Use an immersion blender or transfer the soup to a blender, and blend until smooth.

5. Season with salt and pepper to taste.

6. Serve hot, garnished with a dollop of plain yogurt, fresh cilantro, and toasted pumpkin seeds if desired.

20.Mango Avocado Salad

Ingredients:

- 4 cups mixed salad greens

- 1 ripe mango, peeled and diced

- 1 ripe avocado, peeled and diced

- 1/4 cup red onion, thinly sliced

- 1/4 cup chopped fresh cilantro

- 1/4 cup toasted cashews or almonds

- 2 tablespoons extra virgin olive oil

- 1 tablespoon lime juice

- Salt and pepper to taste

Instructions:

1. In a large bowl, combine mixed salad greens, diced mango, diced avocado, thinly sliced red onion, chopped fresh cilantro, and toasted cashews or almonds.

2. In a small bowl, whisk together extra virgin olive oil, lime juice, salt, and pepper to make the dressing.

3. Drizzle the dressing over the salad and toss gently to coat.

4. Serve immediately as a refreshing and flavorful salad option.

21.Lentil and Vegetable Soup

Ingredients:

- 1 cup dried green lentils, rinsed
- 4 cups vegetable broth
- 1 onion, diced
- 2 carrots, diced
- 2 celery stalks, diced
- 2 cloves garlic, minced
- 1 teaspoon ground cumin
- 1 teaspoon paprika
- 1/2 teaspoon dried thyme
- Salt and pepper to taste
- 2 cups chopped spinach or kale
- Juice of 1 lemon
- Optional: chopped fresh parsley for garnish

Instructions:

1. In a large pot, combine dried green lentils and vegetable broth. Bring to a boil, then reduce heat and simmer for 15-20 minutes or until lentils are tender.

2. In the meantime, heat olive oil in a skillet over medium heat. Add diced onion, diced carrots, diced celery, and minced garlic. Sauté until vegetables are softened.

3. Add sautéed vegetables to the pot of lentils. Stir in ground cumin, paprika, dried thyme, salt, and pepper.

4. Add chopped spinach or kale to the pot and simmer for an additional 5 minutes until greens are wilted.

5. Stir in lemon juice and adjust seasoning if necessary.

6. Serve hot, garnished with chopped fresh parsley if desired.

22. Almond Butter Banana Smoothie

Ingredients:

- 1 ripe banana

- 2 tablespoons almond butter

- 1 cup unsweetened almond milk

- 1 tablespoon honey or maple syrup (optional)

- 1/2 teaspoon vanilla extract

- Ice cubes

Instructions:

1. In a blender, combine ripe banana, almond butter, unsweetened almond milk, honey or maple syrup if using, vanilla extract, and ice cubes.

2. Blend until smooth and creamy.

3. Pour into glasses and serve immediately as a delicious and satisfying smoothie option.

23.Grilled Lemon Garlic Chicken

Ingredients:

- 4 boneless, skinless chicken breasts
- 2 tablespoons olive oil
- 2 cloves garlic, minced
- Zest and juice of 1 lemon
- 1 teaspoon dried oregano
- Salt and pepper to taste
- Optional: chopped fresh parsley for garnish

Instructions:

1. In a small bowl, whisk together olive oil, minced garlic, lemon zest, lemon juice, dried oregano, salt, and pepper to make the marinade.

2. Place chicken breasts in a shallow dish or resealable plastic bag. Pour the marinade over the chicken, making sure it's evenly coated. Marinate in the refrigerator for at least 30 minutes, or up to 4 hours.

3. Preheat grill to medium-high heat. Remove chicken from marinade and discard excess marinade.

4. Grill chicken breasts for 6-8 minutes per side, or until cooked through and juices run clear.

5. Remove from grill and let rest for a few minutes before serving.

6. Garnish with chopped fresh parsley if desired before serving.

24. Quinoa Black Bean Stuffed Sweet Potatoes

Ingredients:

- 4 medium sweet potatoes
- 1 cup cooked quinoa
- 1 cup cooked black beans
- 1 avocado, diced
- 1/4 cup diced red onion
- 1/4 cup chopped fresh cilantro
- Juice of 1 lime
- Salt and pepper to taste

Instructions:

1. Preheat the oven to 400°F (200°C). Pierce sweet potatoes several times with a fork and place them on a baking sheet lined with parchment paper.

2. Bake sweet potatoes for 45-60 minutes, or until tender.

3. In a large bowl, combine cooked quinoa, cooked black beans, diced avocado, diced red onion, chopped fresh cilantro, lime juice, salt, and pepper. Mix well.

4. Once sweet potatoes are cooked, slice them open lengthwise and fluff the insides with a fork.

5. Stuff each sweet potato with the quinoa black bean mixture.

6. Serve hot as a nutritious and satisfying meal option.

25. Mediterranean Chickpea and Farro Salad

Ingredients:

- 1 cup farro, rinsed

- 2 cups water or vegetable broth

- 1 can (15 ounces) chickpeas, drained and rinsed

- 1 cucumber, diced

- 1 bell pepper, diced

- 1/4 cup red onion, finely chopped

- 1/4 cup Kalamata olives, sliced

- 1/4 cup crumbled feta cheese
- 2 tablespoons chopped fresh parsley
- 2 tablespoons extra virgin olive oil
- 1 tablespoon lemon juice
- 1 teaspoon dried oregano
- Salt and pepper to taste

Instructions:

1. In a saucepan, combine farro and water or vegetable broth. Bring to a boil, then reduce heat, cover, and simmer for 20-25 minutes or until farro is tender. Drain any excess liquid and let it cool.

2. In a large bowl, combine cooked farro, drained and rinsed chickpeas, diced cucumber, diced bell pepper, chopped red onion, sliced Kalamata olives, crumbled feta cheese, and chopped fresh parsley.

3. In a small bowl, whisk together extra virgin olive oil, lemon juice, dried oregano, salt, and pepper to make the dressing.

4. Pour the dressing over the salad and toss gently to coat.

5. Serve chilled or at room temperature as a flavorful and nutritious salad option.

26.Roasted Beet and Goat Cheese Salad

Ingredients:

- 4 medium beets, peeled and diced

- 2 tablespoons olive oil

- Salt and pepper to taste

- 4 cups mixed salad greens

- 1/4 cup crumbled goat cheese

- 1/4 cup chopped walnuts, toasted

- 2 tablespoons balsamic vinegar

- 1 tablespoon honey

- Optional: fresh thyme leaves for garnish

Instructions:

1. Preheat the oven to 400°F (200°C). Line a baking sheet with parchment paper.

2. In a bowl, toss diced beets with olive oil, salt, and pepper until evenly coated.

3. Spread the beets in a single layer on the prepared baking sheet.

4. Roast in the preheated oven for 25-30 minutes or until beets are tender and caramelized, stirring halfway through.

5. In a large bowl, combine mixed salad greens, roasted beets, crumbled goat cheese, and toasted walnuts.

6. In a small bowl, whisk together balsamic vinegar and honey to make the dressing.

7. Drizzle the dressing over the salad and toss gently to coat.

8. Serve immediately, garnished with fresh thyme leaves if desired.

27. Lemon Garlic Shrimp Pasta

Ingredients:

- 8 ounces whole wheat spaghetti or pasta of your choice

- 1 pound large shrimp, peeled and deveined

- 2 tablespoons olive oil

- 4 cloves garlic, minced

- Zest and juice of 1 lemon

- 1/4 teaspoon red pepper flakes (optional)

- Salt and pepper to taste

- 2 tablespoons chopped fresh parsley

- Grated Parmesan cheese for serving

Instructions:

1. Cook pasta according to package instructions until al dente. Drain and set aside.

2. In a large skillet, heat olive oil over medium heat. Add minced garlic and cook for 1-2 minutes until fragrant.

3. Add shrimp to the skillet and cook for 2-3 minutes on each side until pink and cooked through.

4. Stir in lemon zest, lemon juice, red pepper flakes (if using), salt, and pepper.

5. Add cooked pasta to the skillet and toss until well combined and heated through.

6. Remove from heat and stir in chopped fresh parsley.

7. Serve hot, garnished with grated Parmesan cheese.

28.Roasted Vegetable Quiche

Ingredients:

- 1 pie crust (store-bought or homemade)

- 2 cups mixed roasted vegetables (such as bell peppers, zucchini, mushrooms, onions)

- 4 large eggs

- 1 cup milk or half-and-half

- 1 cup shredded cheese (such as cheddar, mozzarella, or Swiss)

- Salt and pepper to taste

- Optional: chopped fresh herbs (such as parsley, thyme, or basil)

Instructions:

1. Preheat the oven to 375°F (190°C). Place the pie crust in a pie dish and crimp the edges.

2. Spread the roasted vegetables evenly over the bottom of the pie crust.

3. In a bowl, whisk together eggs, milk or half-and-half, shredded cheese, salt, and pepper.

4. Pour the egg mixture over the roasted vegetables in the pie crust.

5. Optional: Sprinkle chopped fresh herbs over the top.

6. Bake in the preheated oven for 30-35 minutes or until the quiche is set and golden brown on top.

7. Remove from the oven and let it cool for a few minutes before slicing and serving.

29.Mediterranean Grilled Vegetable Sandwich

Ingredients:

- 1 large eggplant, sliced

- 2 zucchinis, sliced lengthwise

- 1 red bell pepper, halved and deseeded

- 1 yellow bell pepper, halved and deseeded

- 1 red onion, sliced into rounds

- 4 whole grain sandwich buns or ciabatta rolls

- 4 tablespoons hummus

- 2 tablespoons pesto

- 1 cup baby spinach leaves

- Salt and pepper to taste

- Olive oil for grilling

Instructions:

1. Preheat a grill or grill pan over medium-high heat.

2. Brush the eggplant slices, zucchini slices, bell pepper halves, and red onion rounds with olive oil. Season with salt and pepper.

3. Grill the vegetables for 3-4 minutes per side, or until tender and grill marks appear.

4. While the vegetables are grilling, slice the sandwich buns or rolls in half and toast them lightly on the grill.

5. Spread 1 tablespoon of hummus on the bottom half of each bun or roll.

6. Spread 1/2 tablespoon of pesto on the top half of each bun or roll.

7. Layer grilled vegetables and baby spinach leaves on the bottom half of each bun or roll.

8. Close the sandwiches with the top halves of the buns or rolls.

9. Serve warm and enjoy this Mediterranean-inspired grilled vegetable sandwich.

30.Berry Oatmeal Breakfast Bowl

Ingredients:

- 1 cup rolled oats

- 2 cups water or milk of your choice

- 1 cup mixed berries (such as strawberries, blueberries, raspberries)

- 2 tablespoons honey or maple syrup

- 1/4 cup chopped nuts or seeds (such as almonds, walnuts, or pumpkin seeds)

- Optional toppings: sliced banana, shredded coconut, chia seeds

Instructions:

1. In a saucepan, bring water or milk to a boil. Stir in rolled oats and reduce heat to medium-low.

2. Cook oats, stirring occasionally, for 5-7 minutes or until thickened and creamy.

3. Divide cooked oats into serving bowls.

4. Top each bowl with mixed berries, drizzle with honey or maple syrup, and sprinkle with chopped nuts or seeds.

5. Add optional toppings such as sliced banana, shredded coconut, or chia seeds if desired.

6. Serve warm and enjoy this nourishing and delicious berry oatmeal breakfast bowl.

31.Herbed Quinoa Salad

Ingredients:

- 1 cup quinoa, rinsed

- 2 cups water or vegetable broth

- 1 cup cherry tomatoes, halved

- 1 cucumber, diced

- 1/4 cup red onion, finely chopped

- 1/4 cup chopped fresh parsley

- 2 tablespoons chopped fresh mint

- 2 tablespoons extra virgin olive oil

- 1 tablespoon lemon juice

- Salt and pepper to taste

- Optional: crumbled feta cheese

Instructions:

1. In a saucepan, combine quinoa and water or vegetable broth. Bring to a boil, then reduce heat, cover, and simmer for 15-20 minutes or until

quinoa is cooked and liquid is absorbed. Remove from heat and let it cool.

2. In a large bowl, combine cooked quinoa, halved cherry tomatoes, diced cucumber, finely chopped red onion, chopped fresh parsley, and chopped fresh mint.

3. In a small bowl, whisk together extra virgin olive oil, lemon juice, salt, and pepper to make the dressing.

4. Pour the dressing over the quinoa salad and toss gently to coat.

5. Optional: Sprinkle crumbled feta cheese over the salad before serving.

6. Serve chilled or at room temperature as a refreshing and flavorful salad option.

32. Turkey and Vegetable Stir-Fry

Ingredients:

- 1 tablespoon olive oil

- 1 pound turkey breast, thinly sliced

- 2 cups mixed vegetables (such as bell peppers, broccoli, snap peas)

- 2 cloves garlic, minced

- 1 tablespoon grated ginger

- 2 tablespoons low-sodium soy sauce

- 1 tablespoon honey or maple syrup

- 1 tablespoon rice vinegar

- 2 cups cooked brown rice

Instructions:

1. Heat olive oil in a large skillet or wok over medium-high heat.

2. Add thinly sliced turkey breast to the skillet and stir-fry for 3-4 minutes until browned and cooked through. Remove from skillet and set aside.

3. In the same skillet, add mixed vegetables, minced garlic, and grated ginger. Stir-fry for 4-5 minutes until vegetables are crisp-tender.

4. Return cooked turkey breast to the skillet with the vegetables.

5. In a small bowl, whisk together low-sodium soy sauce, honey or maple syrup, and rice vinegar. Pour the sauce over the turkey and vegetables in the skillet.

6. Stir-fry for an additional 1-2 minutes until everything is heated through and coated in the sauce.

7. Serve hot over cooked brown rice.

33.Baked Cod with Lemon and Herbs

Ingredients:

- 4 cod fillets

- 2 tablespoons olive oil

- 2 cloves garlic, minced

- Zest and juice of 1 lemon

- 1 tablespoon chopped fresh parsley

- 1 teaspoon dried thyme

- Salt and pepper to taste

- Lemon wedges for serving

Instructions:

1. Preheat the oven to 400°F (200°C). Line a baking dish with parchment paper.

2. Place the cod fillets in the prepared baking dish.

3. In a small bowl, whisk together olive oil, minced garlic, lemon zest, lemon juice, chopped fresh parsley, dried thyme, salt, and pepper.

4. Pour the mixture over the cod fillets, making sure they are evenly coated.

5. Bake in the preheated oven for 12-15 minutes or until the cod is cooked through and flakes easily with a fork.

6. Serve hot with lemon wedges on the side.

34.Mediterranean Chickpea Wraps

Ingredients:

- 1 can (15 ounces) chickpeas, drained and rinsed

- 1/4 cup diced red onion

- 1/4 cup chopped fresh parsley

- 2 tablespoons lemon juice

- 2 tablespoons extra virgin olive oil

- 1 teaspoon ground cumin

- Salt and pepper to taste

- 4 whole grain wraps or tortillas

- 2 cups mixed salad greens

- 1 cucumber, sliced

- 1/2 cup hummus

Instructions:

1. In a bowl, mash the chickpeas with a fork until slightly chunky.

2. Add diced red onion, chopped fresh parsley, lemon juice, extra virgin olive oil, ground cumin, salt, and

pepper to the mashed chickpeas. Mix well to combine.

3. Warm the wraps or tortillas according to package instructions.

4. Spread a layer of hummus onto each wrap or tortilla.

5. Top with mixed salad greens, sliced cucumber, and a generous scoop of the chickpea mixture.

6. Roll up the wraps tightly and cut in half if desired.

7. Serve immediately or wrap tightly in foil for a portable meal option.

35.Lentil and Vegetable Curry

Ingredients:

- 1 cup dried lentils
- 4 cups vegetable broth
- 1 tablespoon olive oil
- 1 onion, diced
- 2 cloves garlic, minced
- 1 tablespoon grated ginger
- 2 carrots, diced

- 2 potatoes, diced

- 1 can (14 ounces) diced tomatoes

- 1 can (14 ounces) coconut milk

- 2 tablespoons curry powder

- 1 teaspoon ground cumin

- 1 teaspoon ground turmeric

- Salt and pepper to taste

- Fresh cilantro for garnish

- Cooked rice or naan for serving

Instructions:

1. Rinse the dried lentils under cold water.

2. In a saucepan, combine rinsed lentils and vegetable broth. Bring to a boil, then reduce heat, cover, and simmer for 20-25 minutes or until lentils are tender.

3. In a large pot, heat olive oil over medium heat. Add diced onion, minced garlic, and grated ginger. Sauté until softened.

4. Add diced carrots and potatoes to the pot. Cook for 5-7 minutes until slightly softened.

5. Stir in diced tomatoes (with their juices), coconut milk, curry powder, ground cumin, and ground turmeric.

6. Add cooked lentils to the pot and stir to combine. Simmer for an additional 10-15 minutes to allow flavors to meld.

7. Season with salt and pepper to taste.

8. Serve hot over cooked rice or with naan bread, garnished with fresh cilantro.

36. Spinach and Mushroom Quiche

Ingredients:

- 1 pie crust (store-bought or homemade)

- 2 cups fresh spinach leaves

- 1 cup sliced mushrooms

- 1/2 cup diced onion

- 4 large eggs

- 1 cup milk or half-and-half

- 1 cup shredded cheese (such as Swiss, Gruyere, or cheddar)

- Salt and pepper to taste

- Optional: chopped fresh herbs (such as parsley or thyme)

Instructions:

1. Preheat the oven to 375°F (190°C). Place the pie crust in a pie dish and crimp the edges.

2. In a skillet, sauté spinach leaves, sliced mushrooms, and diced onion until spinach is wilted and mushrooms are softened.

3. Spread the sautéed vegetables evenly over the bottom of the pie crust.

4. In a bowl, whisk together eggs, milk or half-and-half, shredded cheese, salt, and pepper.

5. Pour the egg mixture over the vegetables in the pie crust.

6. Optional: Sprinkle chopped fresh herbs over the top.

7. Bake in the preheated oven for 30-35 minutes or until the quiche is set and golden brown on top.

8. Remove from the oven and let it cool for a few minutes before slicing and serving.

37.Mediterranean Chickpea Salad Sandwich

Ingredients:

- 1 can (15 ounces) chickpeas, drained and rinsed

- 1/4 cup diced red onion

- 1/4 cup chopped celery

- 1/4 cup chopped cucumber

- 2 tablespoons chopped fresh parsley

- 2 tablespoons lemon juice

- 2 tablespoons extra virgin olive oil

- Salt and pepper to taste

- 4 whole grain bread slices

- Mixed salad greens

- Sliced tomatoes

- Sliced avocado

Instructions:

1. In a bowl, mash the chickpeas with a fork until slightly chunky.

2. Add diced red onion, chopped celery, chopped cucumber, chopped fresh parsley, lemon juice, extra virgin olive oil, salt, and pepper to the mashed chickpeas. Mix well to combine.

3. Toast the whole grain bread slices if desired.

4. Spread a layer of the chickpea salad mixture onto each bread slice.

5. Top with mixed salad greens, sliced tomatoes, and sliced avocado.

6. Close the sandwiches and serve immediately.

38. Butternut Squash and Apple Soup

Ingredients:

- 1 tablespoon olive oil

- 1 onion, chopped

- 2 cloves garlic, minced

- 1 medium butternut squash, peeled, seeded, and diced

- 2 apples, peeled, cored, and diced

- 4 cups vegetable broth

- 1 teaspoon ground cinnamon

- 1/2 teaspoon ground nutmeg

- Salt and pepper to taste

- Optional toppings: Greek yogurt, chopped chives, toasted pumpkin seeds

Instructions:

1. Heat olive oil in a large pot over medium heat. Add chopped onion and minced garlic, sauté until softened.

2. Add diced butternut squash and diced apples to the pot. Cook for 5-7 minutes until slightly softened.

3. Pour vegetable broth into the pot and bring to a boil. Reduce heat and simmer for 20-25 minutes or until squash and apples are tender.

4. Use an immersion blender to blend the soup until smooth. Alternatively, transfer the soup to a blender and blend in batches until smooth.

5. Stir in ground cinnamon, ground nutmeg, salt, and pepper.

6. Serve hot, garnished with a dollop of Greek yogurt, chopped chives, and toasted pumpkin seeds if desired.

39. Lemon Herb Baked Salmon

Ingredients:

- 4 salmon fillets

- 2 tablespoons olive oil

- Zest and juice of 1 lemon

- 2 cloves garlic, minced

- 1 tablespoon chopped fresh dill

- 1 tablespoon chopped fresh parsley

- Salt and pepper to taste

- Lemon slices for garnish

Instructions:

1. Preheat the oven to 375°F (190°C). Line a baking dish with parchment paper.

2. Place the salmon fillets in the prepared baking dish.

3. In a small bowl, whisk together olive oil, lemon zest, lemon juice, minced garlic, chopped fresh dill, chopped fresh parsley, salt, and pepper.

4. Pour the lemon herb mixture over the salmon fillets, making sure they are evenly coated.

5. Place lemon slices on top of each salmon fillet for extra flavor.

6. Bake in the preheated oven for 12-15 minutes or until salmon is cooked through and flakes easily with a fork.

7. Serve hot, garnished with additional chopped herbs if desired.

40.Quinoa Black Bean Burgers

Ingredients:

- 1 cup cooked quinoa

- 1 can (15 ounces) black beans, drained and rinsed

- 1/2 cup breadcrumbs (whole wheat or gluten-free)

- 1/4 cup diced red onion

- 1/4 cup chopped fresh cilantro

- 1 teaspoon ground cumin

- 1/2 teaspoon smoked paprika

- Salt and pepper to taste

- Olive oil for cooking

- Burger buns and toppings of your choice

Instructions:

1. In a large bowl, mash black beans with a fork until partially mashed.

2. Add cooked quinoa, breadcrumbs, diced red onion, chopped fresh cilantro, ground cumin, smoked paprika, salt, and pepper to the bowl. Mix until well combined.

3. Divide the mixture into 4 equal portions and shape each portion into a patty.

4. Heat olive oil in a skillet over medium heat. Cook the quinoa black bean patties for 3-4 minutes on each side, or until golden brown and heated through.

5. Serve the patties on burger buns with your favorite toppings, such as lettuce, tomato, avocado, and mustard.

41. Caprese Salad with Balsamic Glaze

Ingredients:

- 2 large tomatoes, sliced

- 1 ball fresh mozzarella cheese, sliced

- Fresh basil leaves

- Salt and pepper to taste

- Balsamic glaze for drizzling

Instructions:

1. Arrange tomato slices and mozzarella slices on a serving platter, alternating them.

2. Tuck fresh basil leaves between the tomato and mozzarella slices.

3. Season with salt and pepper to taste.

4. Drizzle balsamic glaze over the salad just before serving.

5. Serve immediately as a refreshing and flavorful salad option.

42. Vegetable Stir-Fried Brown Rice

Ingredients:

- 2 cups cooked brown rice
- 1 tablespoon sesame oil
- 2 cloves garlic, minced
- 1 teaspoon grated ginger
- 1 cup mixed vegetables (such as bell peppers, carrots, snap peas)
- 2 tablespoons low-sodium soy sauce
- 1 tablespoon rice vinegar
- 1 teaspoon honey or maple syrup
- 2 green onions, thinly sliced

Instructions:

1. Heat sesame oil in a large skillet or wok over medium heat.

2. Add minced garlic and grated ginger to the skillet. Sauté for 1-2 minutes until fragrant.

3. Add mixed vegetables to the skillet and stir-fry for 3-4 minutes until crisp-tender.

4. Stir in cooked brown rice and cook for an additional 2-3 minutes to heat through.

5. In a small bowl, whisk together low-sodium soy sauce, rice vinegar, and honey or maple syrup.

6. Pour the sauce over the rice and vegetable mixture. Stir to combine.

7. Cook for another 1-2 minutes until everything is heated through and well coated in the sauce.

8. Remove from heat and garnish with thinly sliced green onions before serving.

43.Turkey and Vegetable Meatballs

Ingredients:

- 1 pound ground turkey

- 1/2 cup grated zucchini

- 1/2 cup grated carrot

- 1/4 cup finely chopped onion

- 2 cloves garlic, minced

- 1/4 cup breadcrumbs

- 1 egg

- 1 tablespoon chopped fresh parsley

- 1 teaspoon dried oregano

- Salt and pepper to taste

- Olive oil for cooking

Instructions:

1. Preheat the oven to 375°F (190°C). Line a baking sheet with parchment paper.

2. In a large bowl, combine ground turkey, grated zucchini, grated carrot, finely chopped onion, minced garlic, breadcrumbs, egg, chopped fresh parsley, dried oregano, salt, and pepper. Mix until well combined.

3. Shape the mixture into meatballs, about 1 inch in diameter, and place them on the prepared baking sheet.

4. Bake in the preheated oven for 20-25 minutes or until meatballs are cooked through and golden brown.

5. Remove from the oven and let them cool slightly before serving.

44. Berry Spinach Smoothie

Ingredients:

- 1 cup spinach leaves

- 1/2 cup mixed berries (such as strawberries, blueberries, raspberries)

- 1 banana

- 1/2 cup plain Greek yogurt

- 1/2 cup unsweetened almond milk or milk of your choice

- 1 tablespoon honey or maple syrup (optional)

- Ice cubes

Instructions:

1. Place spinach leaves, mixed berries, banana, Greek yogurt, almond milk, and honey or maple syrup (if using) in a blender.

2. Add ice cubes to the blender for a colder smoothie.

3. Blend until smooth and creamy.

4. Pour into glasses and serve immediately as a nutritious and refreshing smoothie option.

45.Mediterranean Quinoa Salad

Ingredients:

- 1 cup quinoa, rinsed

- 2 cups water or vegetable broth

- 1 cucumber, diced

- 1 bell pepper, diced

- 1/4 cup red onion, finely chopped

- 1/4 cup Kalamata olives, sliced

- 1/4 cup crumbled feta cheese

- 2 tablespoons chopped fresh parsley

- 2 tablespoons extra virgin olive oil

- 1 tablespoon lemon juice

- 1 teaspoon dried oregano

- Salt and pepper to taste

Instructions:

1. In a saucepan, combine rinsed quinoa and water or vegetable broth. Bring to a boil, then reduce heat, cover, and simmer for 15-20 minutes or until quinoa is cooked and liquid is absorbed. Remove from heat and let it cool.

2. In a large bowl, combine cooked quinoa, diced cucumber, diced bell pepper, finely chopped red

onion, sliced Kalamata olives, crumbled feta cheese, and chopped fresh parsley.

3. In a small bowl, whisk together extra virgin olive oil, lemon juice, dried oregano, salt, and pepper to make the dressing.

4. Pour the dressing over the quinoa salad and toss gently to coat.

5. Serve chilled or at room temperature as a refreshing and flavorful salad option.

46. Chicken and Vegetable Skewers

Ingredients:

- 1 pound boneless, skinless chicken breasts, cut into chunks

- 1 zucchini, sliced

- 1 bell pepper, cut into chunks

- 1 red onion, cut into chunks

- 8-10 cherry tomatoes

- 2 tablespoons olive oil

- 2 cloves garlic, minced

- 1 teaspoon dried oregano

- 1 teaspoon smoked paprika

- Salt and pepper to taste

- Wooden or metal skewers

Instructions:

1. If using wooden skewers, soak them in water for at least 30 minutes to prevent burning.

2. In a bowl, combine olive oil, minced garlic, dried oregano, smoked paprika, salt, and pepper to make the marinade.

3. Thread chicken chunks, sliced zucchini, bell pepper chunks, red onion chunks, and cherry tomatoes onto skewers, alternating the ingredients.

4. Place the skewers in a shallow dish and brush them with the marinade, making sure they are evenly coated. Let them marinate for at least 30 minutes, or up to 4 hours in the refrigerator.

5. Preheat grill to medium-high heat. Grill the skewers for 10-12 minutes, turning occasionally, until chicken is cooked through and vegetables are tender and slightly charred.

6. Serve hot, garnished with chopped fresh parsley if desired.

47.Avocado Tuna Salad

Ingredients:

- 2 cans (5 ounces each) tuna, drained

- 1 ripe avocado, mashed

- 1/4 cup diced red onion

- 1/4 cup diced celery

- 1 tablespoon lemon juice

- 1 tablespoon chopped fresh parsley

- Salt and pepper to taste

- Whole grain bread or lettuce leaves for serving

Instructions:

1. In a bowl, combine drained tuna, mashed avocado, diced red onion, diced celery, lemon juice, chopped fresh parsley, salt, and pepper. Mix until well combined.

2. Serve the avocado tuna salad on whole grain bread slices as a sandwich or on lettuce leaves as lettuce wraps.

3. Enjoy this creamy and flavorful tuna salad as a nutritious meal option.

48. Honey Mustard Glazed Salmon

Ingredients:

- 4 salmon fillets
- 2 tablespoons Dijon mustard
- 1 tablespoon honey
- 1 tablespoon olive oil
- 1 clove garlic, minced
- Salt and pepper to taste
- Lemon wedges for serving

Instructions:

1. Preheat the oven to 400°F (200°C). Line a baking sheet with parchment paper.

2. In a small bowl, whisk together Dijon mustard, honey, olive oil, minced garlic, salt, and pepper to make the glaze.

3. Place the salmon fillets on the prepared baking sheet.

4. Brush the honey mustard glaze evenly over the salmon fillets.

5. Bake in the preheated oven for 12-15 minutes or until salmon is cooked through and flakes easily with a fork.

6. Serve hot with lemon wedges on the side.

49.Quinoa Stuffed Bell Peppers

Ingredients:

- 4 large bell peppers, halved and seeds removed

- 1 cup quinoa, rinsed

- 2 cups vegetable broth

- 1 can (15 ounces) black beans, drained and rinsed

- 1 cup corn kernels (fresh, frozen, or canned)

- 1 cup diced tomatoes

- 1/2 cup diced red onion

- 2 cloves garlic, minced

- 1 teaspoon ground cumin

- 1 teaspoon chili powder

- Salt and pepper to taste

- 1 cup shredded cheese (such as cheddar or Monterey Jack)

- Fresh cilantro for garnish

Instructions:

1. Preheat the oven to 375°F (190°C). Arrange the bell pepper halves in a baking dish.

2. In a saucepan, combine rinsed quinoa and vegetable broth. Bring to a boil, then reduce heat, cover, and simmer for 15-20 minutes or until quinoa is cooked and liquid is absorbed. Remove from heat and let it cool slightly.

3. In a large bowl, combine cooked quinoa, black beans, corn kernels, diced tomatoes, diced red onion, minced garlic, ground cumin, chili powder, salt, and pepper. Mix until well combined.

4. Spoon the quinoa mixture into the bell pepper halves, dividing it evenly among them.

5. Cover the baking dish with foil and bake in the preheated oven for 25-30 minutes or until the bell peppers are tender.

6. Remove the foil, sprinkle shredded cheese over the stuffed bell peppers, and return to the oven. Bake for an additional 5 minutes or until the cheese is melted and bubbly.

7. Serve hot, garnished with fresh cilantro.

50.Mediterranean Lentil Soup

Ingredients:

- 1 cup dried lentils
- 4 cups vegetable broth
- 1 onion, chopped
- 2 carrots, diced
- 2 celery stalks, diced
- 2 cloves garlic, minced
- 1 can (14 ounces) diced tomatoes
- 1 teaspoon dried thyme
- 1 teaspoon dried oregano
- Salt and pepper to taste
- Fresh parsley for garnish
- Lemon wedges for serving

Instructions:

1. Rinse the dried lentils under cold water.

2. In a large pot, combine rinsed lentils, vegetable broth, chopped onion, diced carrots, diced celery, minced garlic, diced tomatoes (with their juices), dried thyme, dried oregano, salt, and pepper.

3. Bring the soup to a boil, then reduce heat, cover, and simmer for 25-30 minutes or until lentils and vegetables are tender.

4. Taste and adjust seasoning with salt and pepper if needed.

5. Ladle the soup into bowls, garnish with fresh parsley, and serve hot with lemon wedges on the side.

51. Mediterranean Chickpea and Spinach Stew

Ingredients:

- 2 tablespoons olive oil

- 1 onion, chopped

- 2 cloves garlic, minced

- 1 teaspoon ground cumin

- 1 teaspoon ground coriander

- 1/2 teaspoon smoked paprika

- 1/4 teaspoon red pepper flakes (optional)

- 1 can (15 ounces) chickpeas, drained and rinsed

- 1 can (14 ounces) diced tomatoes

- 2 cups vegetable broth

- 4 cups fresh spinach leaves

- Salt and pepper to taste

- Fresh parsley for garnish

- Lemon wedges for serving

Instructions:

1. Heat olive oil in a large pot over medium heat. Add chopped onion and minced garlic, sauté until softened.

2. Stir in ground cumin, ground coriander, smoked paprika, and red pepper flakes (if using). Cook for 1-2 minutes until fragrant.

3. Add chickpeas, diced tomatoes (with their juices), and vegetable broth to the pot. Bring to a simmer.

4. Simmer for 15-20 minutes, stirring occasionally, until the stew has thickened slightly.

5. Stir in fresh spinach leaves and cook for an additional 2-3 minutes until wilted.

6. Taste and adjust seasoning with salt and pepper if needed.

7. Serve hot, garnished with fresh parsley and lemon wedges on the side.

52.Roasted Vegetable Quinoa Bowl

Ingredients:

- 1 cup quinoa, rinsed

- 2 cups water or vegetable broth

- 1 sweet potato, peeled and diced

- 1 zucchini, diced

- 1 red bell pepper, diced

- 1 yellow bell pepper, diced

- 1 tablespoon olive oil

- 1 teaspoon dried thyme

- Salt and pepper to taste

- 1 avocado, sliced

- 1/4 cup crumbled feta cheese (optional)

- Lemon wedges for serving

Instructions:

1. Preheat the oven to 400°F (200°C). Line a baking sheet with parchment paper.

2. In a saucepan, combine rinsed quinoa and water or vegetable broth. Bring to a boil, then reduce heat, cover, and simmer for 15-20 minutes or until quinoa is cooked and liquid is absorbed. Remove from heat and let it cool.

3. Place diced sweet potato, diced zucchini, diced red bell pepper, and diced yellow bell pepper on the prepared baking sheet.

4. Drizzle olive oil over the vegetables and sprinkle with dried thyme, salt, and pepper. Toss to coat evenly.

5. Roast in the preheated oven for 20-25 minutes, stirring halfway through, until vegetables are tender and slightly caramelized.

6. Divide cooked quinoa among serving bowls. Top with roasted vegetables, sliced avocado, and crumbled feta cheese (if using).

7. Serve hot or at room temperature, with lemon wedges on the side for squeezing over the bowl.

53. Turmeric Ginger Carrot Soup

Ingredients:

- 1 tablespoon olive oil

- 1 onion, chopped

- 2 cloves garlic, minced

- 1 tablespoon grated ginger

- 1 teaspoon ground turmeric

- 1/2 teaspoon ground cumin
- 1/4 teaspoon ground cinnamon
- 4 cups diced carrots
- 4 cups vegetable broth
- 1 can (14 ounces) coconut milk
- Salt and pepper to taste
- Fresh cilantro for garnish

Instructions:

1. Heat olive oil in a large pot over medium heat. Add chopped onion and sauté until softened.

2. Stir in minced garlic, grated ginger, ground turmeric, ground cumin, and ground cinnamon. Cook for 1-2 minutes until fragrant.

3. Add diced carrots and vegetable broth to the pot. Bring to a boil, then reduce heat and simmer for 15-20 minutes or until carrots are tender.

4. Use an immersion blender to blend the soup until smooth. Alternatively, transfer the soup to a blender and blend in batches until smooth.

5. Stir in coconut milk and simmer for an additional 5 minutes.

6. Taste and adjust seasoning with salt and pepper if needed.

7. Serve hot, garnished with fresh cilantro.

54.Greek Yogurt Parfait

Ingredients:

- 1 cup Greek yogurt

- 1/2 cup granola

- 1/2 cup mixed berries (such as strawberries, blueberries, raspberries)

- 1 tablespoon honey or maple syrup (optional)

- Fresh mint leaves for garnish

Instructions:

1. In a glass or bowl, layer Greek yogurt, granola, and mixed berries.

2. Drizzle honey or maple syrup (if using) over the top for added sweetness.

3. Garnish with fresh mint leaves.

4. Serve immediately as a nutritious and satisfying breakfast or snack option.

55.Cucumber and Avocado Gazpacho

Ingredients:

- 2 large cucumbers, peeled and chopped

- 1 ripe avocado, peeled and diced

- 1/4 cup chopped red onion

- 1 clove garlic, minced

- 2 tablespoons chopped fresh cilantro

- 2 tablespoons lime juice

- 1 cup vegetable broth

- Salt and pepper to taste

- Optional toppings: diced tomato, diced bell pepper, chopped fresh parsley

Instructions:

1. In a blender, combine chopped cucumbers, diced avocado, chopped red onion, minced garlic, chopped fresh cilantro, lime juice, and vegetable broth.

2. Blend until smooth and creamy, adding more vegetable broth if needed to reach desired consistency.

3. Season with salt and pepper to taste.

4. Chill the gazpacho in the refrigerator for at least 30 minutes before serving.

5. Serve cold, garnished with optional toppings such as diced tomato, diced bell pepper, and chopped fresh parsley.

56. Baked Sweet Potato Fries

Ingredients:

- 2 large sweet potatoes, peeled and cut into fries
- 2 tablespoons olive oil
- 1 teaspoon smoked paprika
- 1/2 teaspoon garlic powder
- 1/2 teaspoon onion powder
- 1/2 teaspoon ground cumin
- Salt and pepper to taste
- Optional: chopped fresh parsley for garnish

Instructions:

1. Preheat the oven to 425°F (220°C). Line a baking sheet with parchment paper.

2. In a large bowl, toss sweet potato fries with olive oil, smoked paprika, garlic powder, onion powder, ground cumin, salt, and pepper until evenly coated.

3. Spread the seasoned sweet potato fries in a single layer on the prepared baking sheet, making sure they are not overcrowded.

4. Bake in the preheated oven for 20-25 minutes, flipping halfway through, until fries are golden brown and crispy.

5. Remove from the oven and let them cool for a few minutes before serving.

6. Garnish with chopped fresh parsley if desired.

7. Serve hot as a nutritious and flavorful side dish or snack option.

57.Berry Chia Seed Pudding

Ingredients:

- 1/4 cup chia seeds

- 1 cup unsweetened almond milk or milk of your choice

- 1 tablespoon honey or maple syrup (optional)

- 1/2 teaspoon vanilla extract

- 1/2 cup mixed berries (such as strawberries, blueberries, raspberries)

- Optional toppings: additional mixed berries, sliced almonds, shredded coconut

Instructions:

1. In a bowl or jar, combine chia seeds, unsweetened almond milk, honey or maple syrup (if using), and vanilla extract. Stir well to combine.

2. Cover and refrigerate the chia seed mixture for at least 2 hours or overnight, allowing it to thicken and set.

3. Before serving, stir the chia seed pudding to ensure it's well mixed.

4. Layer the chia seed pudding with mixed berries in serving glasses or jars.

5. Garnish with additional mixed berries, sliced almonds, and shredded coconut if desired.

6. Serve chilled as a nutritious and satisfying dessert or breakfast option.

58.Coconut Curry Lentil Soup

Ingredients:

- 1 tablespoon coconut oil

- 1 onion, diced

- 2 cloves garlic, minced

- 1 tablespoon grated ginger

- 1 tablespoon curry powder

- 1 teaspoon ground turmeric

- 1 cup dried red lentils

- 4 cups vegetable broth

- 1 can (14 ounces) coconut milk

- 2 cups chopped spinach or kale

- Salt and pepper to taste

- Fresh cilantro for garnish

- Cooked rice or naan for serving

Instructions:

1. In a large pot, heat coconut oil over medium heat. Add diced onion, minced garlic, and grated ginger. Sauté until softened.

2. Stir in curry powder and ground turmeric. Cook for 1-2 minutes until fragrant.

3. Add dried red lentils and vegetable broth to the pot. Bring to a boil, then reduce heat and simmer for 15-20 minutes or until lentils are cooked and tender.

4. Stir in coconut milk and chopped spinach or kale. Simmer for an additional 5 minutes.

5. Season with salt and pepper to taste.

6. Serve hot, garnished with fresh cilantro, and accompanied by cooked rice or naan bread.

59.Spinach and Feta Stuffed Portobello Mushrooms

Ingredients:

- 4 large portobello mushrooms, stems removed

- 2 cups fresh spinach leaves

- 1/2 cup crumbled feta cheese

- 1/4 cup chopped sun-dried tomatoes

- 2 cloves garlic, minced

- 2 tablespoons olive oil

- Salt and pepper to taste

- Balsamic glaze for drizzling

Instructions:

1. Preheat the oven to 375°F (190°C). Line a baking sheet with parchment paper.

2. Place portobello mushrooms on the prepared baking sheet, gill side up.

3. In a skillet, heat olive oil over medium heat. Add minced garlic and cook for 1 minute until fragrant.

4. Add fresh spinach leaves to the skillet and cook until wilted.

5. Stir in crumbled feta cheese and chopped sun-dried tomatoes. Cook for an additional 1-2 minutes until heated through.

6. Season with salt and pepper to taste.

7. Divide the spinach and feta mixture among the portobello mushrooms, filling each cap.

8. Bake in the preheated oven for 15-20 minutes or until mushrooms are tender.

9. Drizzle with balsamic glaze before serving.

60.Lentil and Vegetable Curry

Ingredients:

- 1 tablespoon vegetable oil

- 1 onion, chopped

- 2 cloves garlic, minced

- 1 tablespoon grated ginger

- 2 tablespoons curry powder

- 1 teaspoon ground cumin

- 1 teaspoon ground coriander

- 1 cup dried green or brown lentils, rinsed

- 3 cups vegetable broth

- 1 can (14 ounces) diced tomatoes

- 2 cups chopped mixed vegetables (such as carrots, bell peppers, zucchini)

- Salt and pepper to taste

- Fresh cilantro for garnish

- Cooked rice or naan for serving

Instructions:

1. Heat vegetable oil in a large pot over medium heat. Add chopped onion, minced garlic, and grated ginger. Sauté until softened.

2. Stir in curry powder, ground cumin, and ground coriander. Cook for 1-2 minutes until fragrant.

3. Add dried lentils, vegetable broth, and diced tomatoes (with their juices) to the pot. Bring to a boil, then reduce heat and simmer for 20-25 minutes or until lentils are tender.

4. Stir in chopped mixed vegetables and simmer for an additional 10-15 minutes or until vegetables are cooked to your liking.

5. Season with salt and pepper to taste.

6. Serve hot, garnished with fresh cilantro, and accompanied by cooked rice or naan bread.

61.Apple Cinnamon Baked Oatmeal

Ingredients:

- 2 cups old-fashioned oats

- 1 teaspoon baking powder

- 1 teaspoon ground cinnamon

- 1/4 teaspoon salt

- 2 cups unsweetened almond milk or milk of your choice

- 1/4 cup maple syrup or honey

- 1 teaspoon vanilla extract

- 1 apple, peeled and diced

- 1/4 cup chopped nuts (such as walnuts or almonds)

- Optional toppings: Greek yogurt, additional diced apple, drizzle of maple syrup

Instructions:

1. Preheat the oven to 350°F (175°C). Grease a baking dish with cooking spray or butter.

2. In a large bowl, combine old-fashioned oats, baking powder, ground cinnamon, and salt.

3. In a separate bowl, whisk together unsweetened almond milk, maple syrup or honey, and vanilla extract.

4. Pour the wet ingredients into the bowl with the dry ingredients and mix until well combined.

5. Stir in diced apple and chopped nuts.

6. Transfer the oatmeal mixture to the prepared baking dish and spread it out evenly.

7. Bake in the preheated oven for 35-40 minutes or until the top is golden brown and the oatmeal is set.

8. Serve warm, topped with Greek yogurt, additional diced apple, and a drizzle of maple syrup if desired.

62.Lemon Garlic Roasted Broccoli

Ingredients:

- 4 cups broccoli florets

- 2 tablespoons olive oil

- 2 cloves garlic, minced

- Zest of 1 lemon

- Juice of 1/2 lemon

- Salt and pepper to taste

- Grated Parmesan cheese for garnish (optional)

Instructions:

1. Preheat the oven to 425°F (220°C). Line a baking sheet with parchment paper.

2. In a large bowl, toss broccoli florets with olive oil, minced garlic, lemon zest, lemon juice, salt, and pepper until evenly coated.

3. Spread the seasoned broccoli florets in a single layer on the prepared baking sheet.

4. Roast in the preheated oven for 15-20 minutes, stirring halfway through, until broccoli is tender and slightly caramelized.

5. Remove from the oven and sprinkle with grated Parmesan cheese if desired.

6. Serve hot as a nutritious and flavorful side dish.

63. Chocolate Banana Smoothie

Ingredients:

- 1 ripe banana

- 1 tablespoon unsweetened cocoa powder

- 1 tablespoon almond butter or peanut butter

- 1 cup unsweetened almond milk or milk of your choice

- 1/2 cup Greek yogurt

- 1 tablespoon honey or maple syrup (optional)

- Ice cubes

Instructions:

1. Place ripe banana, unsweetened cocoa powder, almond butter or peanut butter, unsweetened almond milk, Greek yogurt, and honey or maple syrup (if using) in a blender.

2. Add ice cubes to the blender for a colder smoothie.

3. Blend until smooth and creamy.

4. Pour into glasses and serve immediately as a delicious and satisfying smoothie option.

64.Grilled Vegetable Quinoa Salad

Ingredients:

- 1 cup quinoa, rinsed

- 2 cups water or vegetable broth

- 2 zucchinis, sliced lengthwise

- 2 bell peppers, halved and seeded

- 1 red onion, sliced into thick rounds

- 2 tablespoons olive oil

- Salt and pepper to taste

- Juice of 1 lemon

- 2 tablespoons chopped fresh herbs (such as parsley, basil, or mint)

- Optional: crumbled feta cheese or goat cheese

Instructions:

1. In a saucepan, combine rinsed quinoa and water or vegetable broth. Bring to a boil, then reduce heat, cover, and simmer for 15-20 minutes or until quinoa is cooked and liquid is absorbed. Remove from heat and let it cool.

2. Preheat grill or grill pan over medium-high heat.

3. Brush sliced zucchinis, halved bell peppers, and sliced red onion with olive oil. Season with salt and pepper.

4. Grill the vegetables for 3-4 minutes per side, or until charred and tender.

5. Once grilled, chop the vegetables into bite-sized pieces.

6. In a large bowl, combine cooked quinoa and grilled vegetables.

7. Drizzle lemon juice over the salad and sprinkle with chopped fresh herbs. Toss gently to combine.

8. If desired, sprinkle crumbled feta cheese or goat cheese over the salad before serving.

9. Serve warm or at room temperature as a nutritious and flavorful side dish or main course.

65.Creamy Pumpkin Soup

Ingredients:

- 1 tablespoon olive oil

- 1 onion, chopped

- 2 cloves garlic, minced

- 1 can (15 ounces) pumpkin puree

- 4 cups vegetable broth

- 1/2 cup coconut milk

- 1 teaspoon ground cumin

- 1/2 teaspoon ground cinnamon

- Salt and pepper to taste

- Optional toppings: toasted pumpkin seeds, drizzle of coconut milk, chopped fresh herbs

Instructions:

1. In a large pot, heat olive oil over medium heat. Add chopped onion and minced garlic. Sauté until softened.

2. Stir in pumpkin puree, vegetable broth, coconut milk, ground cumin, and ground cinnamon. Bring to a simmer.

3. Simmer for 15-20 minutes, stirring occasionally, to allow the flavors to meld together.

4. Use an immersion blender to blend the soup until smooth. Alternatively, transfer the soup to a blender and blend in batches until smooth.

5. Season with salt and pepper to taste.

6. Serve hot, garnished with toasted pumpkin seeds, a drizzle of coconut milk, and chopped fresh herbs if desired.

66.Turkey and Vegetable Stir-Fry

Ingredients:

- 1 pound turkey breast, thinly sliced

- 2 tablespoons soy sauce

- 1 tablespoon rice vinegar

- 1 tablespoon honey or maple syrup

- 1 tablespoon cornstarch

- 2 tablespoons vegetable oil

- 2 cloves garlic, minced

- 1 tablespoon grated ginger

- 2 cups mixed vegetables (such as bell peppers, broccoli, carrots, snap peas)

- Cooked brown rice for serving

Instructions:

1. In a bowl, whisk together soy sauce, rice vinegar, honey or maple syrup, and cornstarch to make the sauce.

2. Heat vegetable oil in a large skillet or wok over medium-high heat. Add minced garlic and grated ginger. Stir-fry for 1 minute until fragrant.

3. Add thinly sliced turkey breast to the skillet and stir-fry until cooked through.

4. Push the turkey to one side of the skillet and add mixed vegetables to the other side. Stir-fry the vegetables until tender-crisp.

5. Pour the sauce over the turkey and vegetables in the skillet. Stir well to coat everything evenly.

6. Continue to cook for 2-3 minutes, or until the sauce has thickened and everything is heated through.

7. Serve hot over cooked brown rice as a nutritious and flavorful meal option.

67.Blueberry Banana Oat Bars

Ingredients:

- 2 ripe bananas, mashed
- 1/4 cup honey or maple syrup
- 1/4 cup unsweetened applesauce
- 1 teaspoon vanilla extract
- 2 cups old-fashioned oats
- 1 teaspoon ground cinnamon
- 1/2 teaspoon baking powder
- 1/2 cup fresh or frozen blueberries

Instructions:

1. Preheat the oven to 350°F (175°C). Grease a baking dish with cooking spray or butter.

2. In a large bowl, combine mashed bananas, honey or maple syrup, unsweetened applesauce, and vanilla extract.

3. Stir in old-fashioned oats, ground cinnamon, and baking powder until well combined.

4. Gently fold in blueberries.

5. Transfer the mixture to the prepared baking dish and spread it out evenly.

6. Bake in the preheated oven for 25-30 minutes, or until the top is golden brown and the bars are set.

7. Let cool before cutting into bars.

8. Serve as a nutritious and portable snack option.

68. Mediterranean Chickpea Salad

Ingredients:

- 2 cans (15 ounces each) chickpeas, drained and rinsed
- 1 cucumber, diced
- 1 bell pepper, diced
- 1/4 cup red onion, finely chopped
- 1/4 cup Kalamata olives, sliced
- 1/4 cup crumbled feta cheese
- 2 tablespoons chopped fresh parsley
- 2 tablespoons extra virgin olive oil
- 1 tablespoon lemon juice
- 1 teaspoon dried oregano
- Salt and pepper to taste

Instructions:

1. In a large bowl, combine chickpeas, diced cucumber, diced bell pepper, finely chopped red onion, sliced Kalamata olives, crumbled feta cheese, and chopped fresh parsley.

2. In a small bowl, whisk together extra virgin olive oil, lemon juice, dried oregano, salt, and pepper to make the dressing.

3. Pour the dressing over the chickpea salad and toss gently to coat.

4. Serve chilled or at room temperature as a refreshing and flavorful salad option.

69.Lemon Herb Grilled Chicken

Ingredients:

- 4 boneless, skinless chicken breasts

- Zest and juice of 2 lemons

- 2 cloves garlic, minced

- 2 tablespoons chopped fresh herbs (such as parsley, thyme, rosemary)

- 2 tablespoons olive oil

- Salt and pepper to taste

Instructions:

1. In a bowl, combine lemon zest, lemon juice, minced garlic, chopped fresh herbs, olive oil, salt, and pepper to make the marinade.

2. Place chicken breasts in a shallow dish and pour the marinade over them. Turn to coat evenly. Cover and refrigerate for at least 30 minutes, or up to 4 hours.

3. Preheat grill to medium-high heat. Remove chicken breasts from marinade and discard excess marinade.

4. Grill chicken breasts for 6-8 minutes per side, or until cooked through and juices run clear.

5. Serve hot, garnished with additional fresh herbs if desired.

70. Quinoa and Black Bean Stuffed Bell Peppers

Ingredients:

- 4 bell peppers, any color

- 1 cup quinoa, rinsed

- 2 cups vegetable broth

- 1 can (15 ounces) black beans, drained and rinsed

- 1 cup corn kernels (fresh, frozen, or canned)

- 1 cup diced tomatoes

- 1/2 cup diced onion

- 2 cloves garlic, minced

- 1 teaspoon ground cumin

- 1 teaspoon chili powder

- Salt and pepper to taste

- 1 cup shredded cheese (such as cheddar or Monterey Jack)

- Fresh cilantro for garnish

Instructions:

1. Preheat the oven to 375°F (190°C). Cut the tops off the bell peppers and remove the seeds and membranes.

2. In a saucepan, combine rinsed quinoa and vegetable broth. Bring to a boil, then reduce heat, cover, and simmer for 15-20 minutes or until quinoa is cooked and liquid is absorbed. Remove from heat and let it cool slightly.

3. In a large bowl, combine cooked quinoa, black beans, corn kernels, diced tomatoes, diced onion, minced garlic, ground cumin, chili powder, salt, and pepper. Mix until well combined.

4. Spoon the quinoa and black bean mixture into the hollowed-out bell peppers, dividing it evenly among them.

5. Place stuffed bell peppers in a baking dish. Cover the dish with foil and bake in the preheated oven for 25-30 minutes.

6. Remove the foil, sprinkle shredded cheese over the stuffed bell peppers, and return to the oven. Bake

for an additional 5 minutes or until the cheese is melted and bubbly.

7. Serve hot, garnished with fresh cilantro.

71. Berry Spinach Salad with Balsamic Vinaigrette

Ingredients:

- 4 cups baby spinach leaves

- 1 cup mixed berries (such as strawberries, blueberries, raspberries)

- 1/4 cup sliced almonds, toasted

- 1/4 cup crumbled feta cheese

- 2 tablespoons balsamic vinegar

- 1 tablespoon extra virgin olive oil

- 1 teaspoon honey

- Salt and pepper to taste

Instructions:

1. In a large bowl, combine baby spinach leaves, mixed berries, toasted sliced almonds, and crumbled feta cheese.

2. In a small bowl, whisk together balsamic vinegar, extra virgin olive oil, honey, salt, and pepper to make the vinaigrette.

3. Drizzle the vinaigrette over the salad and toss gently to coat.

4. Serve immediately as a refreshing and nutritious salad option.

72. Ginger Turmeric Immune-Boosting Tea

Ingredients:

- 2 cups water

- 1-inch piece of fresh ginger, thinly sliced

- 1 teaspoon ground turmeric

- 1 tablespoon honey or maple syrup (optional)

- Juice of 1/2 lemon

- Pinch of black pepper

Instructions:

1. In a small saucepan, bring water to a simmer.

2. Add thinly sliced fresh ginger, ground turmeric, and a pinch of black pepper to the simmering water.

3. Simmer for 5-7 minutes to allow the flavors to infuse.

4. Remove from heat and strain the tea into cups.

5. Stir in honey or maple syrup (if using) and lemon juice.

6. Serve hot as a soothing and immune-boosting beverage.

73. Coconut Mango Smoothie Bowl

Ingredients:

- 1 ripe mango, peeled and diced

- 1/2 cup coconut milk

- 1/2 cup Greek yogurt

- 1 tablespoon honey or maple syrup (optional)

- 1/2 cup granola

- 1/4 cup shredded coconut

- Sliced banana, berries, or other fruit for topping

Instructions:

1. In a blender, combine diced mango, coconut milk, Greek yogurt, and honey or maple syrup (if using). Blend until smooth.

2. Pour the smoothie into a bowl.

3. Top with granola, shredded coconut, and sliced banana, berries, or other fruit.

4. Serve immediately and enjoy this tropical and refreshing smoothie bowl.

74. Lentil and Sweet Potato Shepherd's Pie

Ingredients:

- 2 cups cooked lentils
- 2 large sweet potatoes, peeled and diced
- 2 tablespoons olive oil
- 1 onion, chopped
- 2 cloves garlic, minced
- 2 carrots, diced
- 2 celery stalks, diced
- 1 cup frozen peas
- 1 teaspoon dried thyme
- 1 teaspoon dried rosemary
- Salt and pepper to taste
- 1 cup vegetable broth

- 2 tablespoons tomato paste

- 1 tablespoon soy sauce or tamari

- 1 tablespoon Worcestershire sauce (optional)

- 1 tablespoon cornstarch mixed with 2 tablespoons water

- Fresh parsley for garnish

Instructions:

1. Preheat the oven to 375°F (190°C).

2. Place diced sweet potatoes in a pot of water and bring to a boil. Cook until tender, about 15 minutes. Drain and set aside.

3. In a large skillet, heat olive oil over medium heat. Add chopped onion and minced garlic, sauté until softened.

4. Add diced carrots and celery to the skillet and cook until they start to soften.

5. Stir in cooked lentils, frozen peas, dried thyme, dried rosemary, salt, and pepper.

6. In a small bowl, whisk together vegetable broth, tomato paste, soy sauce or tamari, and Worcestershire sauce (if using). Pour into the skillet and bring to a simmer.

7. Stir in the cornstarch mixture and cook until the mixture thickens, about 5 minutes.

8. Transfer the lentil and vegetable mixture to a baking dish and spread it out evenly.

9. Mash the cooked sweet potatoes with a fork or potato masher until smooth. Spread the mashed sweet potatoes over the lentil mixture in the baking dish.

10. Bake in the preheated oven for 20-25 minutes, or until the top is golden brown and the filling is bubbly.

11. Serve hot, garnished with fresh parsley.

75.Avocado Chocolate Mousse

Ingredients:

- 2 ripe avocados, peeled and pitted

- 1/4 cup cocoa powder

- 1/4 cup maple syrup or honey

- 1 teaspoon vanilla extract

- Pinch of salt

- Optional toppings: sliced strawberries, shaved dark chocolate, chopped nuts

Instructions:

1. In a blender or food processor, combine peeled and pitted avocados, cocoa powder, maple syrup or honey, vanilla extract, and a pinch of salt.

2. Blend until smooth and creamy, scraping down the sides of the blender or food processor as needed.

3. Transfer the avocado chocolate mousse to serving dishes.

4. Chill in the refrigerator for at least 30 minutes before serving.

5. Serve cold, topped with sliced strawberries, shaved dark chocolate, chopped nuts, or your favorite toppings.

76.Mediterranean Chickpea Wraps

Ingredients:

- 1 can (15 ounces) chickpeas, drained and rinsed

- 1 tablespoon olive oil

- 1 teaspoon ground cumin

- 1/2 teaspoon paprika

- Salt and pepper to taste

- 4 whole wheat or spinach wraps

- 1 cup hummus

- 1 cucumber, thinly sliced

- 1 bell pepper, thinly sliced

- 1/4 cup sliced Kalamata olives

- Fresh parsley for garnish

Instructions:

1. In a skillet, heat olive oil over medium heat. Add drained and rinsed chickpeas, ground cumin, paprika, salt, and pepper. Cook for 5-7 minutes, stirring occasionally, until chickpeas are lightly browned and crispy.

2. Warm the wraps according to package instructions.

3. Spread a generous layer of hummus onto each wrap.

4. Divide cooked chickpeas, sliced cucumber, sliced bell pepper, and sliced Kalamata olives among the wraps.

5. Sprinkle with fresh parsley for garnish.

6. Roll up the wraps tightly, folding in the sides as you go.

7. Slice each wrap in half diagonally and serve.

77. Turmeric Ginger Carrot Soup

Ingredients:

- 1 tablespoon olive oil

- 1 onion, chopped

- 2 cloves garlic, minced

- 1 tablespoon grated ginger

- 1 teaspoon ground turmeric

- 4 cups chopped carrots

- 4 cups vegetable broth

- Salt and pepper to taste

- Coconut milk for garnish (optional)

- Fresh cilantro for garnish

Instructions:

1. In a large pot, heat olive oil over medium heat. Add chopped onion, minced garlic, and grated ginger. Sauté until softened and fragrant.

2. Stir in ground turmeric and cook for 1 minute.

3. Add chopped carrots and vegetable broth to the pot. Bring to a boil, then reduce heat and simmer for 20-25 minutes, or until carrots are tender.

4. Use an immersion blender to blend the soup until smooth. Alternatively, transfer the soup to a blender and blend until smooth.

5. Season with salt and pepper to taste.

6. Serve hot, garnished with a swirl of coconut milk (if using) and fresh cilantro.

78.Grilled Salmon with Lemon Dill Sauce

Ingredients:

- 4 salmon fillets

- Salt and pepper to taste

- 2 tablespoons olive oil

- 1 lemon, sliced

- Fresh dill for garnish

For the Lemon Dill Sauce:

- 1/2 cup Greek yogurt

- Zest and juice of 1 lemon

- 2 tablespoons chopped fresh dill

- 1 clove garlic, minced

- Salt and pepper to taste

Instructions:

1. Preheat the grill to medium-high heat.

2. Season salmon fillets with salt and pepper, then brush both sides with olive oil.

3. Place lemon slices on top of each salmon fillet.

4. Grill the salmon for 4-5 minutes per side, or until cooked through and flaky.

5. While the salmon is grilling, prepare the lemon dill sauce. In a small bowl, combine Greek yogurt, lemon zest, lemon juice, chopped fresh dill, minced garlic, salt, and pepper. Mix until well combined.

6. Serve the grilled salmon hot, garnished with fresh dill and accompanied by the lemon dill sauce.

79.Roasted Brussels Sprouts with Balsamic Glaze

Ingredients:

- 1 pound Brussels sprouts, trimmed and halved

- 2 tablespoons olive oil

- Salt and pepper to taste

- Balsamic glaze for drizzling

Instructions:

1. Preheat the oven to 400°F (200°C). Line a baking sheet with parchment paper.

2. In a large bowl, toss Brussels sprouts with olive oil, salt, and pepper until evenly coated.

3. Spread the Brussels sprouts in a single layer on the prepared baking sheet.

4. Roast in the preheated oven for 20-25 minutes, stirring halfway through, until Brussels sprouts are tender and caramelized.

5. Remove from the oven and drizzle with balsamic glaze before serving.

80.Quinoa Salad with Roasted Vegetables

Ingredients:

- 1 cup quinoa, rinsed

- 2 cups water or vegetable broth

- 2 cups diced mixed vegetables (such as bell peppers, zucchini, cherry tomatoes, red onion)

- 2 tablespoons olive oil

- Salt and pepper to taste

- 1/4 cup chopped fresh herbs (such as parsley, basil, mint)

- Juice of 1 lemon

- Optional: crumbled feta cheese or goat cheese

Instructions:

1. Preheat the oven to 400°F (200°C).

2. In a saucepan, combine rinsed quinoa and water or vegetable broth. Bring to a boil, then reduce heat, cover, and simmer for 15-20 minutes or until quinoa is cooked and liquid is absorbed. Remove from heat and let it cool slightly.

3. Place diced mixed vegetables on a baking sheet. Drizzle with olive oil, and season with salt and pepper. Toss to coat evenly.

4. Roast the vegetables in the preheated oven for 20-25 minutes, or until tender and lightly browned, stirring halfway through.

5. In a large bowl, combine cooked quinoa and roasted vegetables.

6. Stir in chopped fresh herbs and lemon juice. Mix until well combined.

7. If desired, sprinkle with crumbled feta cheese or goat cheese before serving.

8. Serve chilled or at room temperature as a nutritious and flavorful salad option.

81.Apple Cinnamon Baked Oatmeal Cups

Ingredients:

- 2 cups old-fashioned oats
- 1 teaspoon baking powder
- 1 teaspoon ground cinnamon
- 1/4 teaspoon salt
- 1 1/2 cups unsweetened applesauce
- 2 eggs
- 1/4 cup maple syrup or honey

- 1 teaspoon vanilla extract

- 1 apple, peeled and diced

- Optional toppings: Greek yogurt, additional diced apple, drizzle of maple syrup

Instructions:

1. Preheat the oven to 350°F (175°C). Grease a muffin tin with cooking spray or line with paper liners.

2. In a large bowl, combine old-fashioned oats, baking powder, ground cinnamon, and salt.

3. In another bowl, whisk together unsweetened applesauce, eggs, maple syrup or honey, and vanilla extract.

4. Pour the wet ingredients into the bowl with the dry ingredients and mix until well combined.

5. Fold in diced apple.

6. Divide the mixture evenly among the muffin cups, filling each about three-quarters full.

7. Bake in the preheated oven for 25-30 minutes, or until the tops are golden brown and a toothpick inserted into the center comes out clean.

8. Let the oatmeal cups cool in the muffin tin for a few minutes before transferring to a wire rack to cool completely.

9. Serve warm or at room temperature, topped with Greek yogurt, additional diced apple, and a drizzle of maple syrup if desired.

== THE END ==

Thank you for choosing our book! We trust that it met or exceeded your expectations.

If you enjoyed our book, kindly consider sharing your thoughts in a review on social media. Your feedback is invaluable as it aids us in enhancing our products and services for future readers.

We sincerely appreciate your support and extend our best wishes to you.